My Grandma is a
∴ Cancer Fighting Queen ∵

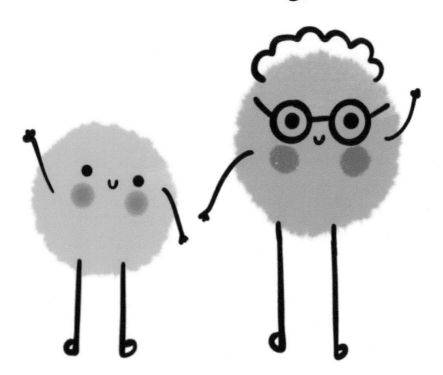

Written and illustrated
by Chelsey Gomez, a
2x cancer survivor.

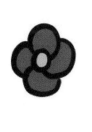

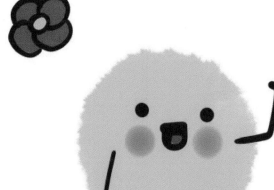

This is my grandma's house.
Yes, the one with the mailbox that looks like a tiny mouse!

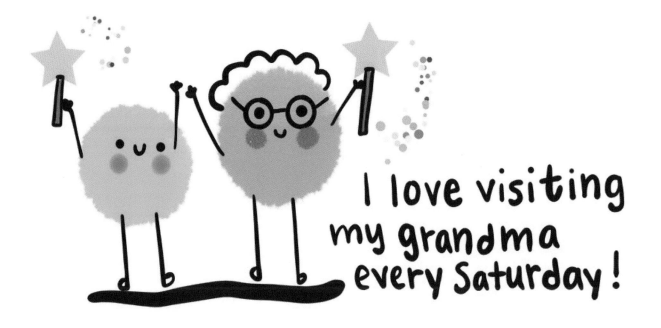

I love visiting my grandma every Saturday!

we have so much fun and
PLAY
PLAY
PLAY!

one of our favorite things to do is baking.

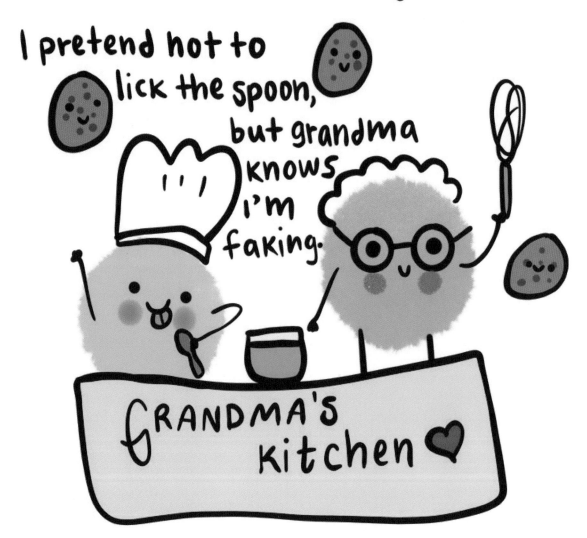

I pretend not to lick the spoon, but grandma knows I'm faking.

GRANDMA'S kitchen ♥

My grandma's house
is my happy place.
I never want to leave
her warm embrace.

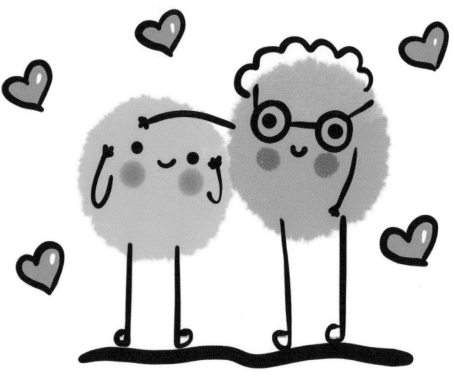

Last Saturday I grabbed Teddy and got ready to go. When I asked if we were leaving soon, my dad said NO.

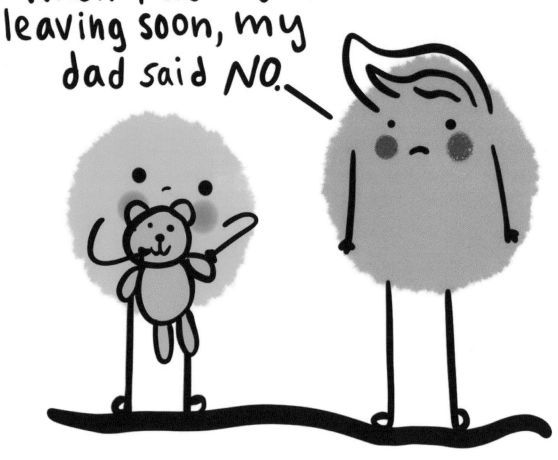

Later I saw my mom and she was sad.
She was crying and talking to my dad.

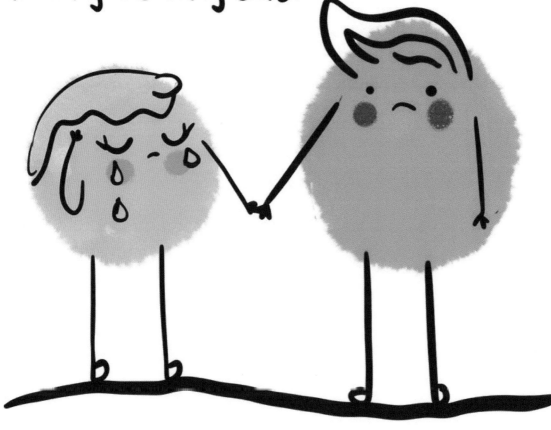

Why are things so different now?
I want to ask why,
but I don't know how.

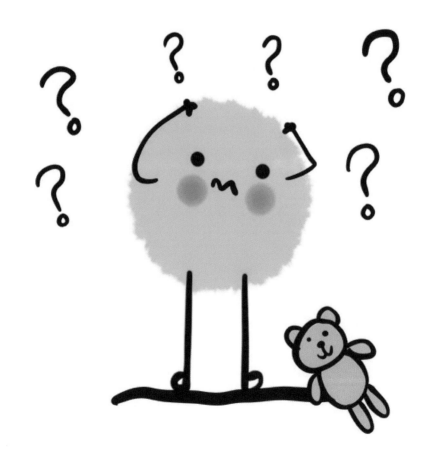

I decided to be brave
and ask mom for an answer.
She told me,
"Grandma has cancer."

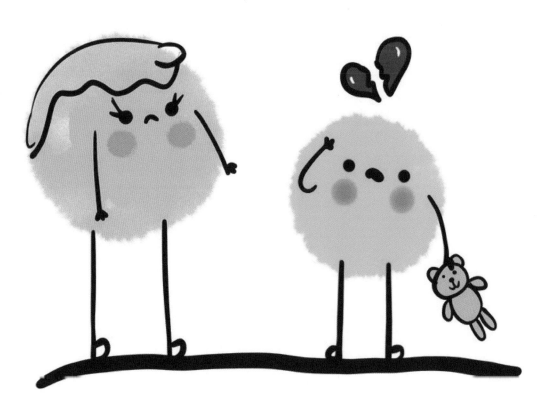

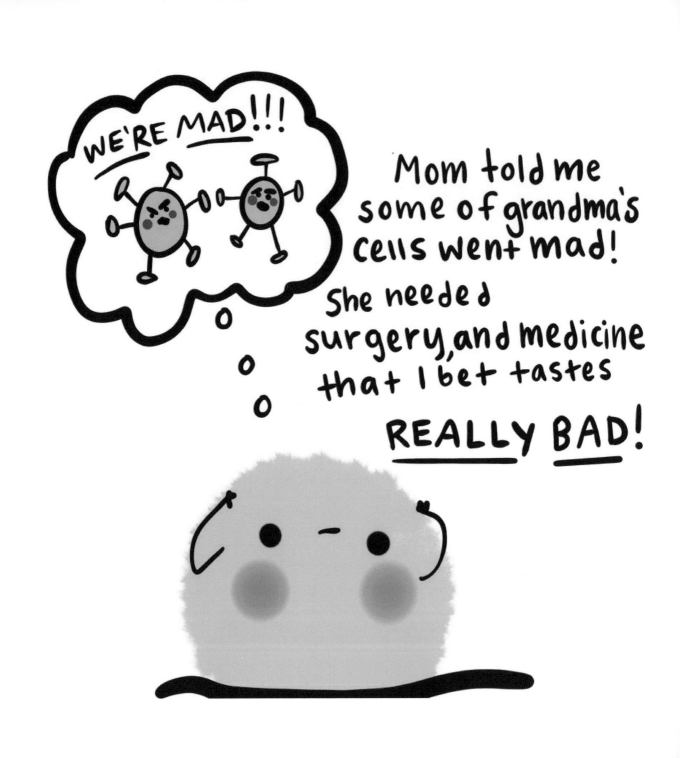

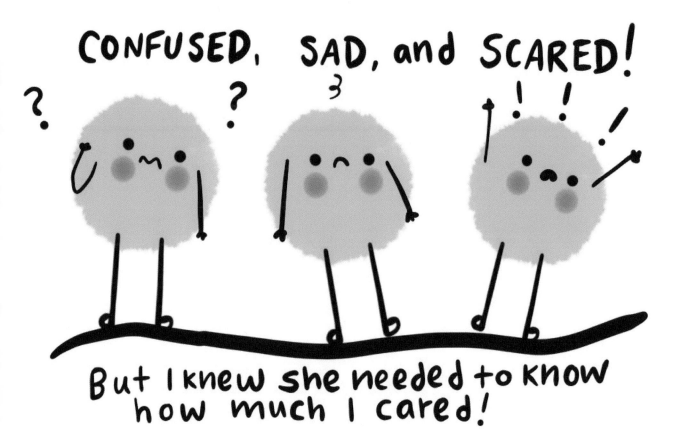

I decided to write her a letter. I just knew it would make her feel better!

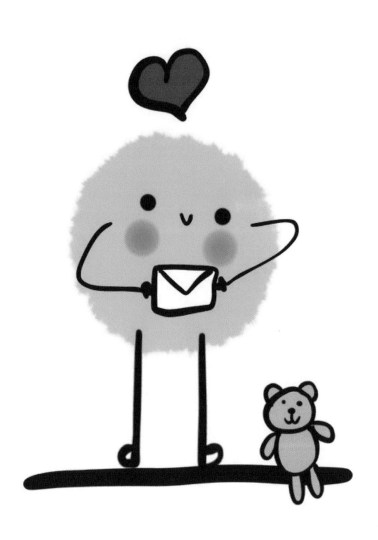

The following Saturday
I was SO EXCITED!
My mom was headed to see
grandma and I was invited!

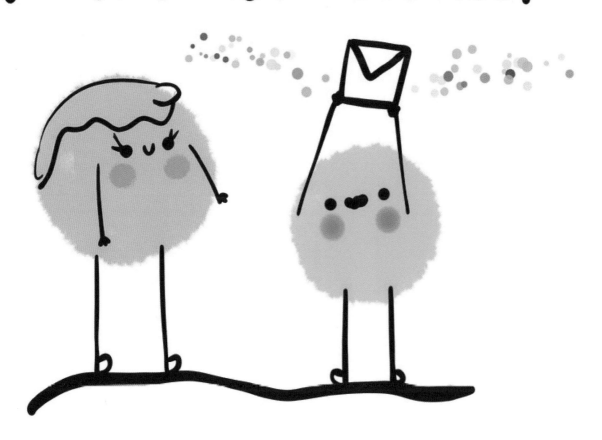

When we arrived I felt butterflies in my tummy.

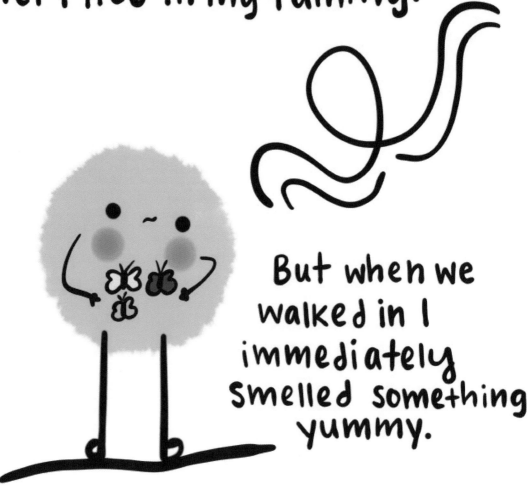

But when we walked in I immediately smelled something yummy.

I saw grandma holding a
cookie and milk in my favorite mug.
I ran to give her a big hug!

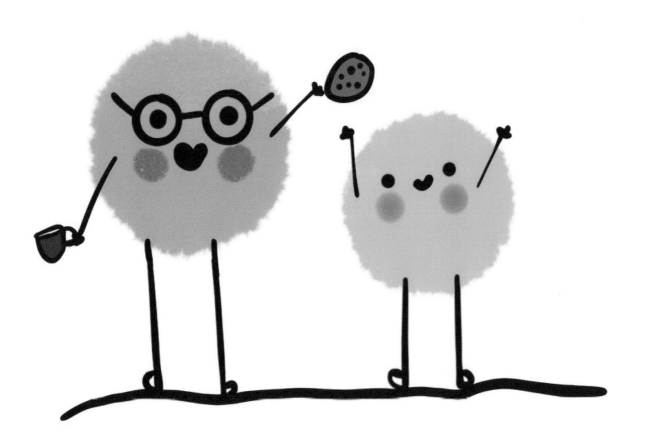

I was so happy to be there, I hardly noticed that grandma lost all her hair!

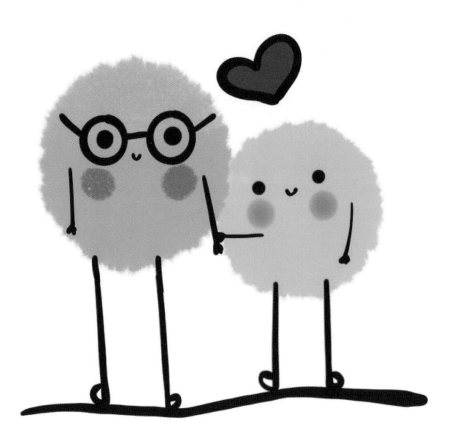

Grandma explained the yucky medicine made her hair fall out. She said it was worth it to get the bad cells out!

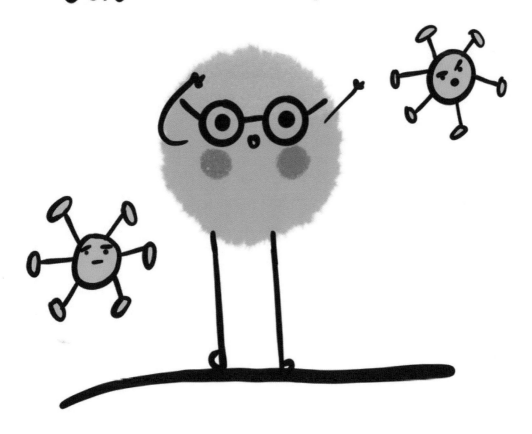

I gave my grandma her card. She read it and then hugged me hard. She was so proud and asked if I would read it out loud.

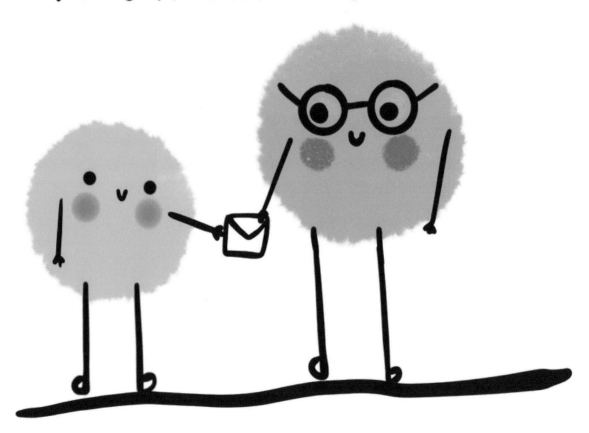

GRANDMA,
your house is my
- HAPPY PLACE -
along with your
♥ warm embrace! ♥
I am sorry you are sick
and I hope you feel
better quick!
cancer might be mean,
but you're a cancer
fighting ♛ QUEEN!
I love you!
(ps. - I'm proud of you
too!)
- PUFF

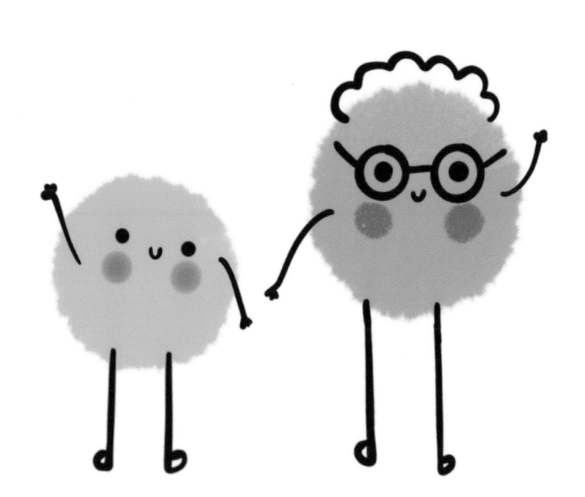

Printed in Great Britain
by Amazon